The Institute of Biology's
Studies in Biology no. 26

Natural History of Infectious Disease

by J. A. Boycott M.A., D.M.

Edward Arnold

First published 1971
by Edward Arnold (Publishers) Limited,
41 Maddox Street,
London, W1R oAN

Boards edition ISBN: o 7131 2303 6
Paper edition ISBN: o 7131 2304 4

Printed in Great Britain by
William Clowes and Sons Ltd, London, Beccles and Colchester

General Preface to the Series

It is no longer possible for one textbook to cover the whole field of Biology and to remain sufficiently up to date. At the same time students at school, and indeed those in their first year at universities, must be contemporary in their biological outlook and know where the most important developments are taking place.

The Biological Education Committee, set up jointly by the Royal Society and the Institute of Biology, is sponsoring, therefore, the production of a series of booklets dealing with limited biological topics in which recent progress has been most rapid and important.

A feature of the series is that the booklets indicate as clearly as possible the methods that have been employed in elucidating the problems with which they deal. Wherever appropriate there are suggestions for practical work for the student. To ensure that each booklet is kept up to date, comments and questions about the contents may be sent to the author or the Institute.

INSTITUTE OF BIOLOGY
41 Queen's Gate
London, S.W.7

Preface

Infectious disease, whether in man or animals or plants, is the result of the invasion of the host by a parasite. For obvious reasons it is infectious disease in man which has had most attention; its detection, treatment and prevention. This is a part of the science and art of medicine and finds no place in this book. Fundamentally the phenomena of infectious disease do not differ in any essential way from those of any other host-parasite relationship. The parasite gains access to the host, draws its nourishment from that source and, usually, passes on to a fresh host. The result of this relationship is some deviation from the normal well-being of the host which may range from trivial to fatal. Throughout our lives we are in contact either continuously or sporadically with parasites which may cause such disturbance in our health. The purpose of this book is to describe some of the factors responsible for the phenomena of infectious disease.

1971   J.A.B.

Contents

'The microbe is so very small
You cannot make him out at all,
But many sanguine people hope
To see him through a microscope.
. . . .
Oh! let us never, never doubt
What nobody is sure about.'

I hope that those who read this book will pay attention to the last lines of
Belloc's verse. The study of infectious disease asks far more questions than
it answers. An experimental approach using man has obvious limitations.
Much has been learned from experiments on animals but these must be
interpreted with caution. No one has yet produced measles or whooping
cough in any experimental animal as we see these diseases in man. It is a
field where argument from analogy is always dangerous and sometimes
misleading. I apologize to all readers for the frequency of 'perhaps' and
'possibly' in these pages but except by using these qualifications I see no
way of making a reasonably connected story.

Infectious disease in man is caused by parasitic animals or plants which
are derived, directly or indirectly, from human or, more rarely, animal
sources. With a few exceptions man does not acquire infectious disease
from animals other than mammals but many arthropods may act as agents
which transmit disease, as, for instance, the mosquito which transmits
malaria or the louse which carries typhus fever. Many parasites associated
with human disease will survive in water or dust for a limited time but all
are ultimately from human or animal hosts.

The parasites may be:
   (i) bacteria,
  (ii) viruses,
 (iii) fungi,
  (iv) protozoa,
   (v) worms (helminths).

In temperate climates worms and helminths play only a small part in causing human disease. Both classes of parasite show such a variety of morpho-
logy and habits that it is difficult to generalize about them and they will be
considered in this book only as illustrations of some of the phenomena of
parasitism.

Bacteria are unicellular plants. They may be rod-shaped (bacilli), spiral
rods (vibrios) or more or less spherical (cocci) and their largest dimensions

lie between 1–10 microns. They are, therefore, visible with the optical microscope. They multiply by binary fission but, unlike the higher plants, the individual cells enlarge only enough to double their size after fission. It is usual to speak of bacterial 'growth' but this means not the enlargement of the individual cell but the multiplication of a colony of identical cells. One or two of these cells may be enough to establish the parasite in the host but within the host there will be an enlarging colony of several thousand or million bacteria. Such colonial growth may be easily demonstrated *in vitro* and the appearance of these 'colonies' is one of the criteria by which bacterial species are identified. All the bacteria which cause disease in man require organic sources of carbon and nitrogen for multiplication. Most can be grown *in vitro* on chemically defined media but their existence under

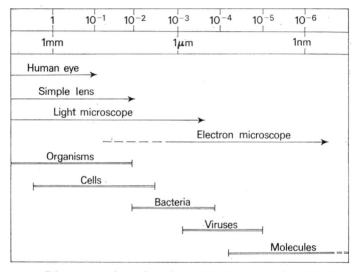

Fig. 1–1   Diagram to show the relationship between a logarithmic scale, the means of observation and the structures which can be resolved. (From Dodge, *An Atlas of Biological Ultrastructure*, Edward Arnold, 1968.)

these artificial conditions can bear only a rough and ready relation to their lives as parasites within the host. Most parasitic bacteria require an adequate supply of oxygen for survival which in their parasitic life in the tissues they derive from the blood supply of the host. A few species (e.g. the tetanus bacillus), however, will not grow in the presence of oxygen and will multiply in the host only where no oxygen is available. Most parasitic bacteria grow most rapidly at the body temperature of the host (37 °C in man) but will survive at lower temperatures when they multiply more slowly. A few species are able to resist extremes of heat and cold by assuming a 'spore form' which does not multiply until it reverts to the normal vegetative form when the temperature and moisture of its environment are suitable. Except for these all bacteria are killed by exposure to 45 °C for a few minutes. Some species of bacteria are provided with flagella which give them limited powers of motility but the importance of these is unknown. In others the bacterial cell is surrounded by a mucoid capsule which plays some part in protecting them, especially within their host. Pathogenic bacteria owe their ability to enter the tissues of the host and to damage the tissues to the production of toxins which occurs only when the cells are multiplying briskly. Some of these toxins (endotoxins) are closely linked to the bacterial cell and appear to operate only in its immediate vicinity but others (exotoxins) produce their damage in sites far removed from the place where the bacteria are multiplying. Infection with the diphtheria bacillus is limited to the throat but its toxin can produce serious damage to the muscle of the heart. There has been much argument about the nature of bacterial toxins but it is enough to say that they have many of the characters of enzymes. Some toxins have been isolated and identified. Each appears to have a specific destructive action on some element of the host's tissues: haemolysin breaks up the red cells, and lecithinase hydrolyses the lecithin which is incorporated in cell membranes. Some exotoxins will survive temperatures which are fatal to the bacteria which produce them. One of these, the toxin formed by *Clostridium botulinum* is, weight for weight, the most poisonous substance known.

The fungi which are parasitic on man are unicellular or multicellular plants and most are rather larger than bacteria. Yeasts and yeast-like fungi are usually seen as single round cells which multiply by producing small 'buds'. When detached from the parent these grow to the same size. The filamentous fungi (moulds) have branching threads which produce a tangle of intertwined hyphae visible to the naked eye (as may be seen on the surface of some home-made jam). Reproductive bodies develop on these filaments which repeat the cycle in a suitable environment. Some species show an elementary sexual process. The individual organism, in contrast to a bacterium, increases in size but 'growth' as usually understood is local multiplication. Little is known of fungal toxins but in general the parasitic life of fungi is not very different from that of bacteria.

The viruses are transmissible particulate entities which multiply only within the cells of the host. They vary much in size and may not be a homogeneous group of parasites. The diameter of the virus of psittacosis, a disease of birds occasionally transmitted to man, is 300 mμ (1 mμ = 0·000 001 mm) and its volume about 1000 times greater than that of the virus of poliomyelitis (diameter 28 mμ). The difference in size is about the same as that between a guinea-pig and a cow. The smallest viruses are not much larger than the largest protein molecules. The viral cell has a central core of nucleic acid which is DNA in some species and RNA in others. This core is covered by an envelope of protein which serves to protect it while the cell is outside the host, gives each species of virus its distinguishing characteristics and provides the enzymes which assist the penetration of the host. Within the host only the nucleic acid is concerned in multiplication, the materials for which are provided by the host cell. Before the infective particles are discharged by the host—which may be an immediate or gradual process—they develop a fresh protein envelope. The effects of viruses on their host and the reactions of the host to their presence are similar to those of bacteria. It has been postulated that viruses are, in fact, highly specialized bacteria adapted to an intracellular life.

1.1   A note on the names of parasites

All parasites have Linnaean binomials. In this book it will usually be enough to name their genera or, more often, the disease with which they are commonly associated. For example, the genus *Streptococcus* contains *Str. viridans*, *Str. haemolyticus*, etc. but they will all be named as streptococci. Diphtheria is caused by *Corynebacterium diphtheriae* but throughout is termed the diphtheria bacillus.

Parasites and Disease 2

2.1 The smaller parasites of man

Parasitism is a state of metabolic dependence. The parasite depends upon the host, completely or partially, for its essential nutriments, either for all or for a part of its life. In addition the host may afford the parasite shelter or transport. What distinguishes the pathogenic parasites (i.e. those which cause disease) from others is that their presence in the host provokes a reaction by the host. The man who suffers from dysentery is not aware of the millions of dysentery bacilli in his bowel but of the diarrhoea which they cause. It is this reaction to the presence of the parasites which we call infectious disease.

There are many bacterial and fungal parasites in the human body which persist there for an indefinite time without causing any obvious sign of ill-health. They are commensal or symbiotic parasites. There are the bacteria (Dubos' 'autochthonous bacteria') which live in close association with the inner wall of the stomach. Their numbers remain constant in health and disease and the part that they play in our life is unknown. None is implicated in causing ill-health. In contrast to these the skin, the mouth, the large bowel and the vagina each has its characteristic bacterial flora. In health the kinds and number of the bacteria in these sites remain constant but disease, disturbances of metabolism and antibiotic drugs will alter the flora qualitatively and quantitatively. These bacteria are commonly regarded as the 'natural' flora of the body. It will be noticed that all the parts of the body where they are found are open to or in connection with the outside air. The tissues of the body, the muscles, the liver, kidneys, brain and blood are normally sterile, i.e. entirely free of parasites. The part played by the normal flora in our lives is uncertain. By a monopoly of the available nutriment or some other form of competition it may help to prevent the invasion of the body by pathogenic parasites. If the normal flora of the large bowel is destroyed by an antibiotic drug the bowel is liable to be invaded by bacteria capable of causing disease. It has been shown that some of the bacteria normally living in the bowel can synthesize some vitamins *in vitro*. Many vegetarian diets appear to be deficient in vitamins but the users show no sign of this deficiency. It is probable that their needs are made up by bacterial activity in their bowels. Whatever their functions the bacteria which make up the natural flora show one characteristic very relevant to the cause of disease. If these bacteria gain entry into a part of the body other than their natural habitat they may become pathogenic. The commonest cause of infections of the urinary tract is *Escherichia coli* which is the predominant member of the normal flora of the large bowel. Excluding the autochthonous bacteria all or almost all the symbiotic and commensal bacteria found in man can be the cause of disease in certain circumstances. The rigid distinction often made between pathogenic and non-pathogenic bacteria is really meaningless. Some bacteria when established in the body almost always cause disease, others do so very rarely but the distinction is statistical and not absolute. We carry many millions of staphylococci on our skin which produce disease only when an accident—such as a nick when shaving—introduces them into the sterile tissues beneath the skin to produce a pimple. The gonococcus, after causing an acute attack of gonorrhoea, may persist in the body without producing any obvious signs of the disease until it has the opportunity to spread to a fresh victim. This ability of some bacteria to linger in the tissues is of some practical importance. The patient who has recovered from diphtheria or typhoid fever may continue to harbour the causative organism for months or years. They do him no harm but are a real danger to the rest of the community. Such a 'carrier' was Typhoid Mary, a cook who moving from one employer to another was responsible for at least seven outbreaks of this disease.

Much less is known of the 'natural' occurrence of viruses in the body because most of those which have been studied in detail are those responsible for recognized diseases of man or animals. From time to time, however, viruses have been isolated more or less by chance which cannot be assigned as the cause of any known disease, the so-called 'orphan viruses'. Some pathogenic viruses having got a foothold in the body remain there for life appearing as a cause of disease only when the resistance of the body is weakened by some other infection. An example is the herpes virus which causes a crop of small pustules round the mouth and nose whenever the victim suffers a severe cold.

Because they multiply so rapidly within the host, the number of bacteria, fungi or viruses which gain access to the body is of less importance than the number of such parasites as worms. A worm enters the body in its larval or adult form incapable of further multiplication whereas, if the environment is suitable, 10 bacteria may increase to 1 million within a few hours. For any one of the smaller parasites, however, there is a minimum number below which infection is unlikely but of the details of this little is known.

It has been shown that the dose of tubercle bacilli necessary to cause disease in guinea-pigs (which are exceptionally susceptible animals) is about 1 bacillus but 1000 or more staphylococci must be introduced into the skin to make infection certain.

2.2 The nature of disease

No definition of disease will satisfy everyone. A man with tonsillitis is likely to have a body temperature above normal (37 °C), a sore throat and a headache: he feels poorly and goes to bed. A man with tuberculosis of the lungs may make no complaint at all except of a chronic cough and of bodily weakness which does not prevent him from doing sedentary work. The man with tonsillitis will be quite well within a few days whereas the man with tuberculosis will die of it if he receives no treatment. One man will make light of discomforts which would send another to bed whether these be due to a twisted ankle, an infectious fever or intense unhappiness. Looked at in this light disease might be defined as a condition of body or mind which prevents a man from earning his daily bread but such a definition, though useful to the lawyer or administrator, is not of much value in the study of the natural history of infectious disease. For this purpose 'disease' must be limited to the effects produced by parasites in the human host and demonstrable objectively either in life or by examination of the body *post mortem*. Whether the patient feels ill is largely irrelevant.

Infectious disease differs from all other diseases in one important way. The doctor can know if a patient's heart is failing by observing his circulation and the results of taking exercise: he uses only his five senses and accumulated experience. A broken leg can be diagnosed by feeling it and studying an X-ray photograph but on this evidence alone it is impossible to say if the patient has fallen downstairs or been hit by a car. In the diagnosis of the parasitic diseases it is almost always possible to detect not only the changes in the body caused by the parasite but also the parasite itself. Bacteria and fungi can be seen with the microscope and grown *in vitro*: it is by the character of their growth *in vitro* and their biochemical activities that one species is commonly distinguished from another. A few viruses have a shape so characteristic that they may be identified under the electron microscope but most are detected by their ability to grow in tissue culture, i.e. in living cells from man or animals growing *in vitro*. Protozoa and worms are usually identified by microscopic appearance alone. Most pathogenic worms are visible to the naked eye but their eggs on which their detection often depends must be sought with a microscope. It is in the detection of the parasite that the laboratory has a part to play but, as often as not, its function is only to confirm the doctor's suspicion.

The finding of a parasite is not, by itself, enough to establish beyond doubt that the patient's illness is caused by that parasite. To make the doctor's diagnosis reasonably certain he will take into account the whole state of the patient, his recent history, his symptoms and his signs. (Symptoms are what the patient feels as, for example, a headache. Signs are what the doctor discovers by examining him; that his temperature is above normal, or the glands in his neck are swollen.)

The doctor is unlikely to search the whole body at random to discover a parasite. If the patient has a sore throat he will look for bacteria or viruses in the throat; if he has diarrhoea he will do the same in the faeces. Experience tells him that certain parasites are associated with certain changes in the body and he will concentrate his search on these.

In the male the gonococcus gives rise to a discharge from the penis. If the patient has had sexual intercourse within the last few days the doctor has good reasons for thinking that he has gonorrhoea. Gonorrhoea may take a mild or a severe form but experience tells the doctor that it is unlikely that the patient's signs and symptoms are caused by any parasite other than the gonococcus. The doctor can, however, be certain of his diagnosis only when the gonococcus is detected in the discharge. When transmitted to a fresh host the gonococcus will always cause gonorrhoea and will never give rise to acne or tonsillitis. This is an example of a *specific* infection just as the typhoid bacillus always gives rise to typhoid fever and the poliovirus to poliomyelitis. Most of the early knowledge of human parasites was derived from the study of specific infections caused by a distinctive parasite which gave rise to a characteristic disease in the patient. Because this experience has taught us how to prevent or avoid these diseases specific infections such as typhoid fever or diphtheria or poliomyelitis are now rare in Great Britain.

In contrast to these are the *non-specific* infections. A wound of the skin caused by a fall in the road opens the tissues (which are normally free from bacteria) to any bacteria which happen to be on the victim's skin, on his clothes or in the dirt of the road. There may be one kind of bacterium or many but, irrespective of their kind, they will multiply in the wound to produce the same effects, pain, swelling and a discharge of pus. The doctor who examines the patient can have no grounds for suspecting that any one species of bacterium is responsible for the infection. It may be any one out of many. Experience tells him that some species of bacteria are likely to cause a more severe infection than others but until the bacteria in the wound have been identified in the laboratory he must be content to treat 'an infected wound' and not a specific infection. If the bacteria happen to spread to another patient the disease which they cause may be quite different from that in the first: different in the part of the body affected, different in signs and symptoms and different in outcome. These non-specific infections, especially of grazes and wounds, are one of the major problems of medicine today and especially in those who are elderly or ill from some other cause which makes them more susceptible to infection (see p. 26).

2.3 The cause of infectious disease

An infectious disease is one caused by a parasite which every so often leaves its host to establish itself in another. Infection is the process by which it becomes established in the new host. This property, infectivity, must be distinguished from virulence which is the ability to provoke a reaction in the host.

The parasite which is perfectly adapted to its host uses it only as a source of nourishment and provokes no reaction to its presence. The autochthonous bacteria in the stomach are examples of these. The pathogenic parasite, however, stimulates its host to react in some way to its presence and it is the more obvious of these reactions which are the signs and symptoms of disease. A high temperature, coughing and diarrhoea are all examples of these reactions. Except for a few large parasites such as tapeworms which can be seen with the naked eye we are aware that we harbour parasites only by the reactions which they cause. These reactions will be considered in detail at a later stage but since they all appear to be directed to the expulsion of the parasite or the neutralization of its effects they are to its disadvantage. If the reaction of the host is feeble the parasite will continue to thrive or even to spread. The parasite which succeeds so well that it kills its host does itself no good however: it alters its environment so that it may be unable to survive and makes its escape from the dead host a matter of difficulty. (Contrary to popular opinion dead men shed few parasites.) The reaction produced by most of our pathogenic parasites is only sufficient to make their stay in the host a temporary one and to force them to seek a fresh host from time to time. They are, in fact, disorderly lodgers who are always getting notice to quit. The more acute the reaction which the parasite causes the more often it must move to a fresh host. The immediate effects of acute tonsillitis are severe and painful but the disease is short-lived. The first reaction to tuberculosis is milder (though the damage caused to the body will, in the end, be far more serious) but the disease may last for years. Coughing, sneezing and diarrhoea are all common reactions to infection which assist in the expulsion of the parasite. A few parasites (such as *Brucella abortus* which causes undulant fever) establish themselves deep in the tissues of the human host and can seldom escape even after death. Their parasitic life comes to an end.

The smaller parasites cannot move to a fresh host by their own efforts. It is true that some bacteria have organs of locomotion (flagella) but it is unlikely that the ability to move a few metres in water is of much value in finding a host. The purpose of these organs seems rather to allow the bacterium to seek the environment most suitable for survival. Coughing sets free the parasites of the respiratory tract enclosed in minute droplets of mucus and saliva. These are so small (50–200 microns in diameter) that they remain suspended in the air for some time. How far and how fast they travel will clearly depend on the vigour of the cough and the air currents in the room but they are subject to continual dilution by clean air. Some of these droplets will fall to the ground and be incorporated in the dust and this again may be spread by draughts or domestic cleaning with a broom. (A vacuum cleaner will also spread dust unless it sucks it into a paper bag which can be destroyed.) There has been much argument whether a book which has been read by someone suffering from an infectious disease may be a source of infection to those who read it later. The risk is probably a slight one but some doctors disinfect all books from such a source. The major difficulty is that, as with many other things which may have been used by the infectious patient, adequate disinfection is likely to be destructive. Clothes and bed-clothes are especially likely to be infected by coughing but are easily cleaned and disinfected. In civilized communities the parasites expelled by diarrhoea are disposed of in the sewage works but elsewhere are always likely to contaminate food and drinking water. Even in this country the risk of this is not negligible. Many bacteria from the human bowel can survive and even multiply in water so that if they gain access to flowing water, either a natural stream or a main pipe, they may spread far. This is, of course, equally true if contaminated water gains access to foodstuffs. One large outbreak of typhoid fever was spread by milk which had been contaminated by the water, used to rinse the churns, which was polluted with human faeces. The normal processes of whole-sale and retail trade are likely to spread any parasite which is in the food. Beef, infected by polluted water while being canned in the Argentine, spread typhoid fever in Aberdeen in 1968. Parasites on the skin may be removed by contact or disseminated in the air on the cells of the epidermis which are being shed continually. A biting insect may transfer a parasite that is in the blood stream to its next victim on its proboscis; the limit to this is the flight range of the insect. (Such a mechanical transfer must be distinguished from the process by which malaria is spread. The malarial protozoon shares an active parasitic life between man and mosquito.)

All these means of local spread play a part in the movement of parasites but the most important factor is the movement of the infected host. The man with a cold who stays at home will transmit his infection only to his family and friends. If he enters other houses or public places he will carry his parasites with him. Out of doors he is likely to be a less potent source of infection because his viruses will be diluted in the air. It is not the man who is seriously ill who is the chief source of infection to others but he who, while spreading the parasite, feels well enough to go about his normal duties. In some diseases too the infected person begins to shed his parasites before he feels ill or when he feels quite well again. Mention has been made of Typhoid Mary who was well enough to carry on her avocation of cook while she spread typhoid bacilli intermittently. Such 'carriers' of typhoid fever are not uncommon.

It is the human host who, from time to time, introduces exotic infectious diseases into Great Britain. When all immigrants came to this country by sea the voyage gave time for diseases to be detected before the ship arrived. Travel by air has resulted in the introduction of lethal diseases such as smallpox which have been acquired on the other side of the globe but which have shown their symptoms only after the victim is at large in this country. During the last two centuries cholera has sometimes spread westward from its home in Bengal via Afghanistan and Persia to reach Russia and even Great Britain. Traditionally the disease moved as fast as a man can walk but now that the caravan of camels is a thing of the past the pace is probably that of the lorry which has replaced them. It was not the camels or the goods which they carry which spread the disease but the merchants and their hangers-on.

The Survival of the Parasite   3

Since relatively few human parasites are spread by the direct contact of one host with another it is clear that most of them must be able to survive outside the body of the host for at least a short time. A measure of the mortality likely to occur in this passage from one host to another is the disproportion between the number of parasites discharged by one host and the number necessary to establish infection in another. Whereas the number expelled by an infected host must be measured in millions the number needed to produce infection in another may be less than ten. There are several natural factors which make survival at this stage hazardous and of these the two most important are probably drying and the lethal action of ultra-violet light. Desiccation, especially at low temperatures, is not invariably fatal but reduces the number of living parasites considerably. Most bacteria and fungi survive longer in a damp environment. Bacteria (and probably viruses) are protected to some extent by the saliva or faeces in which they are expelled from the body and some species, such as the tubercle bacillus, will remain viable in dust for some weeks. Bacteria which form spores will survive almost indefinitely under natural conditions. Fungal spores are not so resistant but many fungi will exist in soil or animal excreta for a long time. Poliovirus shed in the faeces can be detected in sewage while smallpox virus remains alive in the scabs of dead skin shed by the patient. There are, however, a few bacteria such as the gonococcus which are so sensitive to drying and cooling that intimate contact of the two hosts is essential for transfer.

It is not only an old wives' tale that sunlight is healthy. Ultra-violet light is bactericidal but has low powers of penetration under natural conditions. It has been used deliberately to kill parasites in the air of classrooms and offices but has not proved very successful as measured by the amount of illness in the rooms which have been treated. In warmer climates the heat of the sun may have some importance in destroying parasites but this can seldom be the case in the British Isles. Nevertheless, except for the fact that most of us spend more time indoors with our fellows, there is no obvious explanation why infectious diseases are usually more common in the winter.

Until the introduction of antibiotics (see p. 13) any attempt to interrupt the parasitic cycle had to be limited to the time when the parasite was in transit from one host to another. Few drugs were known which would destroy the parasite once it had entered the host and these had limited applications; as, for example, the arsenical compounds used for the treatment of syphilis. Heating to a temperature which kills the parasite has been one of the methods most commonly used to destroy the parasite in transit.

The surgeon sterilizes his instruments by boiling them in water or heating them in steam under pressure. The explorer boils his drinking water. Heating is an essential part of the process of canning meat, fruit and vegetables. Most of the milk sold in Great Britain is 'pasteurized', i.e. heated to 161 °F (71·8 °C) for 15 sec. This process kills most bacteria, viruses and fungi without upsetting the complex physico-chemical constitution of milk as does boiling. Pasteurization has made milk-borne disease a rarity and at the same time has given the household milk a longer 'life' by destroying the bacteria which cause it to turn sour.

Only extremes of cold unobtainable except in the laboratory are fatal to bacteria. At temperatures below 10 °C few bacteria (and none of those pathogenic to man) will multiply. The purpose of refrigerating food is not to destroy any bacteria which may be in it but to prevent an increase in their numbers. Since the dose of bacteria received by the host may determine whether any infection results any process which prevents their multiplication in the vehicle of infection will limit their ability to cause disease. It is, however, of more importance in everyday life that refrigeration prevents the multiplication of the bacteria which cause foodstuffs to decay. Few of these are a serious risk to health. 'Bad' food may or may not contain pathogenic bacteria. Because of its taste we do not as a rule eat it but game and cheese are customarily eaten in a state of decay caused by bacteria and no one seems the worse for it. When food is refrigerated it is important that it should be kept cold continually until eaten or cooked. Quite short periods at higher temperatures will allow bacterial multiplication.

Chemical as well as physical methods are used to destroy the parasite outside the host. Certain groups of chemical substances, commonly known as disinfectants or antiseptics, will kill almost all the smaller parasites. Those in common use are alkalis, soaps, phenols and halogens but there are many others. Each of these groups has its advantages and failings: some are very poisonous, some corrosive and some unstable. The efficacy of all is reduced to some extent by the presence of organic matter so that the removal of all dirt by a preliminary washing increases their activity. Most drinking water is disinfected with hypochlorites or gaseous chlorine after the dirt and impurities which are usual in raw water have been removed by precipitation and filtration. Such 'chlorinated' water has made water-borne disease as rare as that transmitted by milk. Before he makes his incision in the skin the surgeon disinfects the site with iodine or some other disinfectant to prevent the infection of the wound by the bacteria living on the skin. The nurse keeps the thermometer in the sickroom in a mild disinfectant to avoid the transfer of bacteria from one mouth to another (but it is wiser to use an individual thermometer for each patient). It must be made clear, however, that the advice to 'kill germs' in the advertisements for disinfectants has its limitations. Some of these disinfectants may be applied to the intact skin without causing harm but none can be used to kill the parasite within its host. Most disinfectants are as poisonous

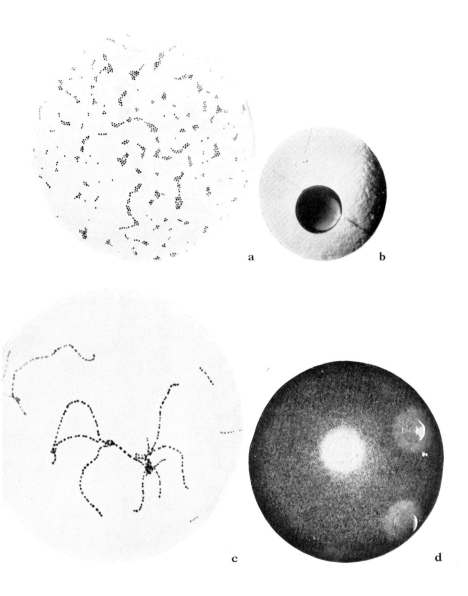

Plate 1 **(a)** *Staphylococcus aureus* cells, × 1000;
(b) *Staph. aureus* colony, × 8;
(c) *Streptococcus pyogenes* cells, × 1000;
(d) *Str. pneumoniae* colony, × 8. (From Topley and Wilson's *Principles of Bacteriology and Immunity* by Wilson, G. S. and Miles, A. A., Edward Arnold, London.)

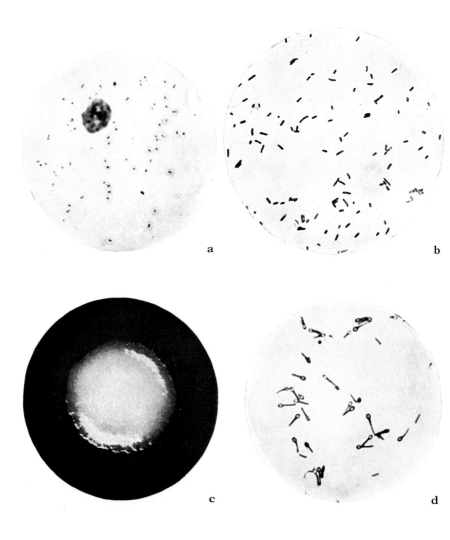

Plate 2 **(a)** *Streptococcus pneumonia* cells and capsules, × 1000;
(b) *Escherichia coli* cells, × 1000;
(c) *E. coli* colony, × 8;
(d) *Clostridium tetani* cells and spores, × 1000. (From Topley and Wilson's *Principle of Bacteriology and Immunity* by Wilson, G. S. and Miles, A. A., Edward Arnold London.)

to man as they are to his parasites and many of them interfere with the natural defences of the body against infection. The ideal disinfectant has yet to be found and disinfectants are certainly used aimlessly and to excess. The many gallons of phenolic emulsion which are slopped round the public lavatories do no more than add a refreshing smell to the air and there is no evidence that such things as 'medicated' toilet paper do anything to prevent the spread of infectious disease. In spite of all reason the out-dated idea that disease is caused by foul smells survives: malaria (= bad air) got its name from the smell of the marshes which bred the mosquitoes which transmit the disease.

Antiseptics and disinfectants must be distinguished from antibiotics. The latter (penicillin, streptomycin, tetracycline, etc.) are, in general, not poisonous to the host but lethal to many of his bacterial parasites. They can therefore be used to break the parasitic cycle at the time when the parasite is within the host and have thereby revolutionized the treatment of infectious disease. Most are biological products of various fungi but a few have been synthesized. Their anti-bacterial activity is semi-specific. A very few antibiotics kill almost all bacteria but the activity of most is limited to only a few bacterial genera. The doctor chooses the antibiotic which is lethal to the bacterial parasite which is responsible for the patient's illness. In general they are not active against viruses.

3.1   The parasite's search for a host

The parasite set free in air or water will have the best opportunity of entering a new host if there are a lot of potential victims at hand. A school classroom or a London tube train offers more chance of finding a host than a private house or an open field. Ventilation has no magical virtues but, as has been said, it dilutes the concentration of parasites in the air. There is good sense in isolating the patient with an infectious disease from his fellows but if isolation is to succeed it must be complete. The inhabitants of such an island as Tristan da Cunha are customarily free of the common infectious diseases until they receive a visit from a passing ship when there is likely to be an epidemic. In the same way a waterborne parasite will do more harm if it gains access to a main water supply than if it is in an isolated spring. Foodborne infection in the home will be limited to members of the household but in a hotel or a canteen it may spread to hundreds. The food may have been contaminated before it entered the kitchen or by those who have cooked or served it if these are carriers of disease or suffering from an infection so mild that it does not prevent them working. Cooking kills most parasites but sometimes the centre of a mass of food such as a large joint of beef never reaches a bactericidal temperature in the process.

A distinction is usually apparent between the rate of spread of a food- or waterborne infection and one derived directly from an infected host. A patient suffering from a streptococcal sore throat is likely to shed his

2—N.H.I.D.

parasites over 3–4 days. The number of his victims will depend on the number of people with whom he has contact and the closeness of his association with them. Furthermore, each of his victims will probably be the source of further infections some days later and so on. The epidemic may last for weeks. In contrast infected food or drink will cause disease in

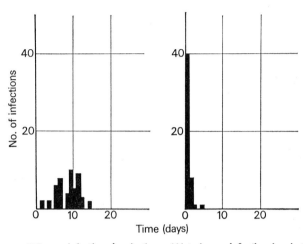

Airborne infection: incubation period approx. 36–48 hr

Waterborne infection: incubation period less than 24 hr

Fig. 3–1 Timetable of airborne and waterborne infections: 50 victims of each.

all or most of those who consume it on the same day, but because the origin of the disease can usually be ascertained the infected foodstuff will not be served a second time. Those who suffer the primary infection may spread the disease further but this is unusual (see Fig. 3–1).

The Defences of the Body against Infection

It is a common error to assume that to bring host and parasite together is enough to establish infection. It is obviously not so. The doctors or nurses who care for the victims of infectious disease seldom catch it: nor does the microbiologist who handles the parasites in the laboratory. It is true that they take simple precautions to avoid infection such as washing their hands but only when dealing with the more dangerous diseases such as smallpox do they take deliberate measures to avoid the parasite. We must all be exposed to airborne parasites discharged by our companions, especially in crowds and in the winter, but for most of us it is an exception and not the rule that we catch a cold or influenza. Even in a school it is most unusual if every pupil in a class or everyone who sleeps in one dormitory catches whatever disease may be prevalent. Experiment has shown that when the cold virus is put deliberately in the nostrils of volunteers not all develop colds. Water- and foodborne parasites may be proportionately more successful than those spread in the air but 100% infection is exceptional. Passage from one host to another seems to be most successful when it depends (as in gonorrhoea) on direct contact of the two but some fungal diseases spread in this way, e.g. 'footrot', fail to infect a large number of those exposed to them.

To produce disease a parasite must be able to enter the body of the host and to reach some part of it where multiplication is possible. This is not a single process but a series of attempts to overcome and penetrate the natural or acquired barriers to parasitic invasion. Each move by the parasite to establish itself provokes counter-measures in the host. These defences of the host are of several kinds, general and local, innate and acquired, but they do not operate independently and it is impossible to define the exact sphere of activity of each separate mechanism. Nor do all the defences act simultaneously but rather as one fails to check the invasion another comes into effect. At any stage in the process the parasite may be checked or destroyed or expelled from the host, or, alternatively, it may establish itself to cause disease or death.

The first barriers to infection are the skin and other integuments of the body. The skin is impervious to most bacteria, fungi and viruses, and it has antiseptic powers, probably because of the fatty acids and soaps secreted by its glands. Streptococci placed on the dry healthy skin disappear after a few hours. It has long been thought that a few species of bacteria such as the anthrax bacillus can pass through the intact skin but infections due to these parasites commonly occur on the hands or other exposed surfaces and few of us are without a few minor scratches there. Even the smallest perforation is enough to allow bacteria to penetrate: for a body the size of a bacterium a needle prick is a wide tunnel. It is not only perforations which will allow bacteria to pass through the skin into the underlying tissues. A burn caused by heat or caustic chemicals also destroys the defences of the skin: the illness caused by a burn is only partly due to the burn itself and much of the damage is due to subsequent bacterial infection.

The eyes lack the tough armour of the skin but are protected by a continual flow of secretion (tears) which wash any bacteria which light on the eye into the lachrymal duct and thence into the nose. In addition the tears contain an enzyme-like substance, lysozyme, which destroys many bacteria. Lysozyme is not, however, active against all micro-organisms and more parasites may enter the body through the eye than is commonly thought.

The mouth has its own indigenous flora which persists with little alteration in spite of the wide variety of organisms which enter the mouth in food or drink. Bacteria tend to stick to the film of mucus which covers the inside of the mouth and are moved backwards by the flow of saliva until they are swallowed. Saliva too contains a bactericidal substance allied to lysozyme. Bacteria in food which do not come into direct contact with the mucus film are swallowed at once. In the stomach they are exposed to the hydrochloric acid secreted there and this is one of the body's most effective defences. Most of the known pathogenic bacteria are killed at pH $3 \cdot 0 - 4 \cdot 0$ and this is probably fatal to most other parasites taken in the food. The protection is not, however, absolute. Some people, naturally or because of disease, secrete no acid in their stomachs or do so only intermittently. It is possible that bulky foods such as porridge shield some bacteria or act as buffers. Some viruses will certainly survive the passage through the stomach: the poliovirus given as a protective vaccine (see p. 25) is administered absorbed on a lump of sugar. The parasite which manages to pass through the stomach may either multiply in the intestine or enter the tissues. The dysentery bacilli are an example of the first, multiplying in the intestine to the point where they may largely replace the normal flora but never penetrating the intestinal wall. The typhoid bacillus on the other hand passes through the intestinal epithelium to be transported through the lymph stream to such organs as the spleen.

The convoluted anatomy of the interior of the nose provides an extensive mucus surface on which dust, bacteria and viruses are trapped. Some of these may invade and multiply in the mucus membrane but most are swept backwards by the cilia on the epithelium to be swallowed or ejected by coughing or sneezing. There is some evidence that invasion by a virus of the respiratory tract facilitates subsequent infection by a bacterium. It is common experience that a cold or influenza is followed immediately by tonsillitis or bronchitis.

Bacterial infection of the vagina is far less common in women of child-bearing age than in younger or older females. At the child-bearing age the healthy vagina has an acid reaction (pH 3·5–4·5) which prevents the multiplication of most pathogenic bacteria. It may be a similar mechanism which prevents the infection of the urinary tract from its open lower end.

It was mentioned above that a burn of the skin is just as liable to admit bacterial parasites as a scratch. Infections of other parts of the body may be due to abnormalities which are physiological rather than anatomical. Anything which interferes with the free flow of urine is liable to lead to infection of the urinary tract: this may be a stone in the bladder or the pressure of the enlarged womb in pregnancy. Complete obstruction of the bowel allows the bacteria which make up the normal flora of the lumen to pass through the wall to infect the peritoneal cavity. The mechanisms responsible for these failures of the normal defensive mechanisms cannot be explained but they emphasize the extent to which freedom from infection depends on the general state of health.

The protection afforded by the skin and the mucus membranes of the respiratory tract and the bowel shelter us from what is probably far more than 99% of the parasites which come into contact with us. Nevertheless, that parasites invade our tissues and thereby cause disease shows that under certain circumstances these defences fail. Some general causes will be described later but it is worth considering what is the property which allows a parasite to establish itself in the throat or the bowel. It is known that some viruses secrete an enzyme which attacks the mucopolysaccharide coating of nasal epithelium. Some viruses have an affinity for a particular tract of epithelium where their enzymes find a suitable substrate. The larval stage of parasitic schistosome worms secrete an enzyme which allows them to penetrate the epithelium of a snail which is their intermediate host. There is little doubt that many parasites have the ability to secrete one or more enzymes which will facilitate their entry into mucus membrane but very little is known of the details of this process. There must be a fundamental difference between the dysentery bacillus which in spite of rapid multiplication remains localized within the lumen of the bowel and the typhoid bacillus which, entering the body by the same route in food or drink, penetrates the bowel wall to establish itself in the tissues of the body.

Once a parasite is within an epithelium cell or has passed this barrier it will begin to multiply provided it can find suitable nutriment. The nutritional needs of the parasite can be satisfied only by the cells and fluids of the host and since the cells of the body are differentiated chemically as well as morphologically a parasite must find the nutritional environment which suits it best (see p. 29). It is probable that every parasite secretes a variety of enzymes and it must be assumed that the enzyme system of the dysentery bacillus, well adapted to draw nourishment from the contents of the bowel, lacks the elements which would allow it to penetrate the bowel wall and obtain its needs from the tissues of the body. In the same way the yeast-like fungi which exist in the vagina live on the secretions of the vagina and do not penetrate the epithelium.

Except for these superficial infections (and the lumen of the bowel must be thought of as outside the tissues of the body) the multiplication of the parasite in the body is followed at once by a series of reactions in the host. Whether the stimulus to these reactions is a toxin or toxins produced by the parasite or the products of the cells of the host damaged by such toxins is unknown. Some reactions are almost specific to the parasite which causes them but many different parasites produce reactions which, if not identical, differ from each other in their extent and severity rather than in their nature. It must be added too that similar reactions may be provoked by irritant substances which are not of biological origin. In some countries the injection of petrol or turpentine under the skin is a method used to avoid compulsory military service. The resulting abscess resembles one caused by staphylococci but, initially at any rate, is free of bacteria.

4.1   The cellular defences

The general pattern of the defensive mechanisms which involve the cells of the host is shown when a bacterial parasite such as a staphylococcus enters the tissues through a recent scratch. The parasite finds itself in the intracellular spaces of the deeper layers of the skin. Here it begins to multiply and in the process produces toxins which destroy the cells in its immediate vicinity. The first reaction of the host to the multiplication of the parasite is a dilatation of the small blood vessels around the site which brings about a local increase in blood supply. (This can be seen as the small area of red skin round a pimple.) The increase in the blood supply has two main effects. The first is to increase the number of the phagocytic leucocytes which circulate in the blood and which have the property of engulfing small particles such as bacteria. Their assembly at the point of infection is mediated by a chemotactic mechanism. The second is an increase in the local concentration of the bactericidal substances normally present in the blood. What these are and how they operate is open to argument. They may be reinforced by other bactericidal substances which are the result of previous infection by the specific parasite (see p. 22). The general result of the local dilatation of the blood vessels is to concentrate rapidly the available defensive mechanisms at the site of infection.

The next reaction of the body is an increase in the permeability of the walls of the dilated blood vessels so that fluid containing both leucocytes and the bactericidal substances passes into the tissues to make direct contact with the bacteria. To this is due the local swelling round an infection. The swelling is often painful because the fluid in the tissues is under pressure. A boil on the nose where there is little room for expansion between skin and bone hurts more than one in a place where there is a soft fatty layer beneath the skin. As the leucocytes accumulate at the site of infection they form the whitish pus (or matter) that can be squeezed from a pimple. Under the microscope pus is seen to consist of leucocytes, bacteria and the fragments of the cells of the host destroyed by the bacterial invasion. Some bacteria are lying free and some have been engulfed by the leucocytes (see Plate 3a).

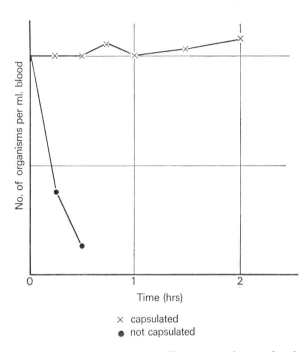

× capsulated
● not capsulated

Fig. 4–1   Protective action of capsules. (Pneumococci, capsulated and not capsulated, injected intravenously into mice. Blood of the mice then sampled every 15 minutes.)

It is possible that these defensive processes are sufficient to check the bacterial invasion. The toxins are neutralized, the bacteria are taken up by the leucocytes and the body replaces the cells which have been destroyed. Most pimples heal without treatment and leave no trace: squeezing them may be amusing but probably interferes with their healing. Some species of bacteria are, however, more invasive than others. It may be that the toxins which they produce are more destructive or that they multiply more rapidly. Some bacteria will multiply inside the leucocyte which engulfs them and 'live to fight another day'. Some can penetrate and multiply inside the tissue cells of the host (as viruses do) and are thereby sheltered in part from the defences of the host. Some species seem to evade the leucocytes and some produce toxins (leucocidins) which destroy the leucocyte. The possession of a capsule seems to protect a bacterium against phagocytosis (see p. 19). There are also many general factors which influence the ability of the host to defend itself (see page 26) and within a single species of host some individuals are by nature more resistant to infection than others.

As the struggle between host and parasite continues the former mobilizes a second kind of phagocytic cell, the macrophage, and lays down a wall of fibrin to fence the site of infection. Fibrin is the substance derived from the blood which causes it to clot when it escapes from a blood vessel. As the area of the infection enlarges the fibrin barrier extends. As the fibrin ages it is replaced by fibrous tissue which can be felt as the hard wall of a boil surrounding a cavity filled with pus. The larger the boil the slower it will heal; if it is close under the skin it is likely to leave a scar caused by the healing and contraction of the fibrous tissue. See Plate 3b.

Staphylococci tend to cause localized infections of this kind. Other species of bacteria may spread far and wide in the tissues unchecked by the local defences of the host. They may overflow into a blood vessel and be carried to other parts of the body to initiate new infections there. They will localize where the nutritional conditions are most suitable. Such disease will often take its name from the site where the parasite multiplies. Meningitis is an infection of the meningeal space immediately outside the central nervous system caused by a parasite carried there in the blood. Endocarditis is a blood-borne infection of the lining of the heart. Both are the end-results of infection introduced from outside the body. Wherever any infection localizes it will, if of more than trivial severity, be accompanied by signs and symptoms general to the whole body, a raised temperature and a feeling of ill-health.

A distinction must be made between acute and chronic infections. Those which have been described are usually short-lived leading to either complete healing or to the death of the host. In contrast such a bacterium as the tubercle bacillus gives rise to an infection which may last for years. The parasite lives for all or a part of the time within the host cells. The infection remains localized in one organ, usually the lungs. It provokes an intense fibrin reaction which may in time distort the anatomy of the lung and make a large part of it incapable of oxygenating the blood. One focus of infection will heal while others in different parts of the lung will spring into activity. It might be said that parasite and host have established a stable symbiotic reaction but, until the introduction of antibiotic drugs, the parasite usually killed the host in the end. This is not the only form a tuberculous infection may assume: in the young it may be rapid blood-spread infection ending fatally within weeks. Leprosy, undulant fever and syphilis may all cause chronic infections marked by a similar balance between host and parasite.

The mechanisms which protect the host against a parasite limited to the lumen of the bowel, such as the dysentery bacillus, are basically the same as those described above. The bowel has a 'normal' bacteriological flora with which the parasite must compete for foodstuffs. If invasion by a pathogenic parasite is successful this normal flora is likely to be overgrown and even replaced by the newcomer but there is evidence which suggests that the normal flora can sometimes prevent the establishment of the fresh parasite. The toxins of the parasite stimulate the musculature of the bowel (causing colic) and provoke the outpouring from the bowel wall of leucocytes and large quantities of tissue fluids derived from the blood. Not only does this fluid carry bactericidal substances (as in tissue infections) but it dilutes the bacterial toxins and washes away both toxins and parasites as a liquid diarrhoea. Indeed the loss of fluid from the bowel may be so great as to cause the death of the host from dehydration.

The reactions of the body to viral infections are similar to but not identical with those caused by bacteria. The portals of entry are much the same. Some such as the common cold (the nose) or warts (the skin) never spread further. Others spread via the blood or lymph to localize in some organ far removed from the place of entry: smallpox enters through the respiratory tract but its effects are seen in the skin and elsewhere; poliomyelitis passes from the intestinal tract to the central nervous system. Wherever the virus multiplies there is a local mobilization of the fluid and cellular defences. We are all aware of the local swelling of the mucus membrane of the nose in the common cold: it is red, swollen and ticklish and it pours out fluid. One defence mechanism against viruses seems to have no exact parallel in bacterial infections. Host cells infected with one virus appear to be resistant to invasion by another virus. The host cell is stimulated to produce a substance, interferon, which prevents the multiplication of almost any other virus at the site.

Reactions to the presence of fungi are various. Some are well-adapted parasites which survive for years in the tissues walled off by a fibrous reaction. Others do not penetrate the integuments but multiply on the surface of the host nourished by the secretions of the epithelium. The acid reaction of the healthy vagina which prevents bacterial infection does not inhibit the growth of some yeast-like fungi (*Candida* spp.) which may flourish there (see p. 17). The increase in the local blood supply in the superficial layers of the skin, as seen in bacterial infections, is demonstrated by the circular red area which characterizes ringworm, a disease which is caused by one of several fungi.

4.2   The humoral defences

It is traditional to distinguish between the cellular defences of the body and the humoral ones. The former have been described already. The latter consist of the substances either natural or acquired, which circulate in the blood and assist in the protection of the body. The distinction between the two is not absolute since humoral factors have some influence on cellular reactions.

Normal blood is to some extent bactericidal but it is hard to decide whether this is an innate quality or due to protective substances resulting from previous exposure to a variety of parasites (see p. 24). More attention has been devoted to those bactericidal substances which develop as the result of infection. It is common knowledge that very few children suffer second attacks of measles or diphtheria. Infection produces some change in the host which prevents its recurrence. Diphtheria is now a rare disease but much of our knowledge of the changes induced by infection has been derived from it. It must be remembered, however, that it is not the bacterial infection itself which damages the body but the exotoxins produced by the

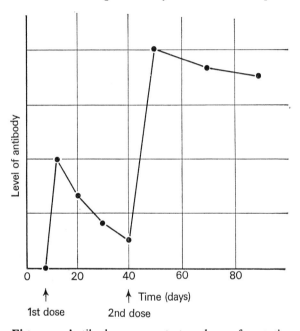

Fig. 4–2   Antibody response to two doses of an antigen.

diphtheria bacillus and acting some way from the site of infection. In this diphtheria differs from most of the common diseases which we meet. It can be shown that in the course of an attack of diphtheria substances are formed which neutralize the toxin and that these circulate in the blood. In more general terms the introduction of a foreign substance (antigen) stimulates the body to produce a globulin (antibody) which reacts specifically with the antigen. The antigen may be a protein, a polysaccharide or even, unusually, a simple substance such as formalin linked to the body's own protein. The essential for an antigen is that it should have a large molecule. Gelatin, a protein with a molecular weight of about 12 000, is a poor antigen; egg-white (molecular weight 40 000) is a good one. Bacterial cells, viruses and bacterial toxins are all effective antigens. Antibodies are globulins with molecular weights 150 000–190 000 which are formed in the lymphoid cells of the body. The reaction of antibody with antigen is always hostile. If the antigen is a bacterium the antibody may agglutinate the bacterial cells to form large clumps which appear to be biologically inactive, or it may render the bacterial cells more sensitive to phagocytosis. In some cases the antibody actually destroys and dissolves the cells. If the antigen is a toxin the antibody will neutralize it. The critical feature of all these reactions is their specificity. Antibody produced in response to diphtheria toxin does not react with or neutralize any other toxin. The antibody provoked by measles virus will not react with any other virus just as an attack of measles does not protect against influenza or chickenpox. The analogy of the key and the lock is not misleading but takes no account of the fact that the antigen-antibody reaction is quantitative. There is an exact and constant relation between any quantity of diphtheria toxin and the amount of antitoxin necessary to neutralize it. The reaction is so delicate that it can be used to distinguish the proteins of two closely related bacteria which appear identical by the cruder methods of organic chemistry.

It can be shown experimentally that the quantity of antibody formed in response to an antigen depends, not only on the amount of antigen, but on whether it is given in one, two or more doses, on the route by which it is given and by the intrinsic ability of the animal to produce it which may vary considerably. Since all biological reactions tend to take place more slowly than purely chemical ones (though, no doubt, they are fundamentally chemical in nature) it may be impossible to detect antibodies until some days after the administration of the antigen. This is important because in the course of an acute infection it is seldom possible to reinforce the antibodies produced by the parasite by giving the host a further dose of the antigen: this will indeed produce antibodies but they will probably be formed too late to be of value. If the antigen is given in two doses the response to the second is likely to be far higher than that caused by the first provided the two doses are separated by some days (see fig. 4-2). An antigen which is slowly released into the tissues is likely to provoke more antibody than the same amount given as a single dose.

Almost from the moment when they can first be detected and whether they are produced by natural infection or artificially the level of antibodies in the body will decline unless there is some further stimulus to their production. The rate at which they decline varies within wide limits. Antitoxins survive for longer than antibodies to bacterial cells or viruses. Antibodies produced by a second dose of the antigen last longer than those provoked by a single dose. Antibody formation occurs relatively quickly compared with the rate at which their level falls. Even a parasite which lives in the lumen of the bowel and never enters the tissues of the body may stimulate the production of detectable antibodies but these are usually at a low level. Some of the bacteria which make up the normal flora of the body produce antibodies in it but it is doubtful if these have any importance.

The antigen-antibody reactions have had much attention because, unlike many of the phenomena described in this book, they lend themselves to experimental study both *in vivo* and *in vitro*. It must not be thought, however, that these reactions alone are responsible for the resistance of the host to a parasite. They reinforce the natural and cellular defences of the body but it is hard to be sure of their relative importance in nature. What is certain is that they give a reasonable explanation of many of the phenomena of infectious disease as it occurs naturally.

Second attacks of measles or diphtheria are rare because the body is protected by antibodies formed during the first attack. Such an immunity to subsequent infections is seen after almost all infectious diseases but its duration varies from for life, as in measles (in most people), to only a few weeks in bacillary dysentery. Common experience would suggest that a cold gives only a short period of immunity but it has been shown that a 'cold' may be caused by several distinct viruses and it is unlikely that the antibodies to any one of these will protect against any other. The duration of artificial immunity varies in the same way. The International Certificates of Vaccination demanded by many countries of all visitors are valid for six months for cholera and three years for smallpox.

It does not follow as a matter of course that if antibodies to a parasite are detectable the host is necessarily immune to the disease. When a patient has had a staphylococcal boil antibodies to staphylococci may be detected but it is notorious that one boil is likely to be followed by another. The level of antibodies produced is not always parallel to the severity of the disease. When exposed to an infectious disease we may acquire it in so trivial a form that we are unaware of our infection: the signs and symptoms depend as much on the host's reaction to the parasite as on the activity of the parasite itself. Nevertheless we may develop antibodies to the parasite and be to some extent immune to a subsequent infection. Antibodies to the mumps virus can be detected in many people who have no recollection of having had the disease and appear to protect these people against later attacks.

Most of us probably have some antibodies to most of the commoner parasites; these may afford us absolute protection or only enough to ensure that we suffer a mild attack. Since these are the result of 'experience' their variety will increase (and perhaps their levels rise) as we get older. Having suffered the 'diseases of childhood'—measles, chickenpox and so on—we are more or less immune in later life. It has been shown that while at the age of 5 years about 20% of children have antibodies to tuberculosis (even among those who have had no close contact with the disease) the proportion has risen to 75% at the age of 15 years. Children from urban homes develop these antibodies quicker than those who live in the country. The newly-born child has had no 'experience' but has acquired antibodies from its mother while *in utero*. In a matter of months these fade but it has been observed that many infectious diseases are uncommon in a child aged less than 12 months. A parasite newly arrived in a community will find no antibodies. When European whalers introduced measles into Fiji in 1875 it killed 25% of the inhabitants but since that date the disease in those islands differs not at all from that seen in Europe. Most of us probably acquire our traces of antibodies in stages. In our early years we pick them up as the result of infections in the family. When we first go to school we come into contact for the first time with parasites which had never entered our home. Then as we mix with more people, go to a new school or perhaps go abroad we add further to our experience of new parasites. These may not produce overt disease but make ready our antibody-forming mechanisms to meet the threat of a second invasion by the parasite. Observation suggests that it is in the first week of term that minor infectious diseases are most common in a school. Antibody levels have declined in the relative isolation of the holidays and a new mixture of potential parasites has been introduced to the school.

Antibodies may be produced deliberately as well as by natural infection. In the last years of the eighteenth century Edward Jenner, a country doctor in Gloucestershire, attributed the immunity of one of his patients to smallpox—then a common and lethal disease in England—to a recent attack of cowpox. Cowpox is a mild natural infection of cattle which is still sometimes transmitted to man. Jenner confirmed his guess by infecting a patient with cowpox and then trying to transfer smallpox to her. He failed, not once but several times. Jenner was a muddle-headed fellow and some of his experiments are unconvincing but essentially he was right. (Incidentally he was the first person to suspect the parasitic habits of the cuckoo—and no one believed him.) He thought that cowpox was a mild form of smallpox but it is now known that these diseases are caused by distinct but closely related viruses. Vaccination (latin *vacca*, a cow) has made smallpox an almost unknown disease in Europe and if applied systematically could do the same in all the world. The same principle has been applied to the prevention of many diseases. The basis of all vaccination is to protect against a dangerous infection either by giving the patient the same disease in a mild form or by giving him an antigen so modified that while it retains the power of producing antibodies it no longer causes any serious damage to the patient. Antigenic overlap such as is shown by cowpox and smallpox is unusual. Against poliomyelitis two vaccines have been used. One consists of a strain of the poliovirus which does not produce disease but which remains antigenic. It is given by the mouth which is the route of natural infection with this virus. (Such non-pathogenic variants of pathogenic parasites are found from time to time by chance or may be produced by long continued cultivation of the parasite *in vitro*.) The other vaccine against poliomyelitis is made of a virulent strain of the virus which has been killed with formaldehyde and is given by injection. Such dead vaccines have been used to protect against both viral and bacterial parasites: examples in common use are those against whooping cough and typhoid fever. In general these killed vaccines are less satisfactory than those which contain a living parasite of weakened virulence which presumably imitate a natural infection more closely. Immunity produced by a killed vaccine is seldom absolute and lasts for a shorter time: it is usually necessary to give two or more doses and these must be injected. The range of parasites against which effective vaccines, live or dead, have been produced is limited. The tubercle bacillus, staphylococci and the gonococcus are all common parasites against which vaccination has been so far impossible, but the reasons for this are obscure.

Vaccination can also be used to protect the host against the exotoxins produced by parasites. Any exotoxin is usually too damaging to be injected into man but after chemical treatment (e.g. with formaldehyde) it loses most of its toxic properties while remaining antigenic. The immunity produced is almost complete and may last from a few years until death. Thirty years ago diphtheria was a killing disease of the young. Now almost all the children in Great Britain receive diphtheria toxoid (i.e. altered toxin) with the result that the disease is virtually unknown. Tetanus toxoid gives almost life-long protection against an uncommon disease with a high mortality.

The antibodies produced artificially resemble the natural ones in almost every way. They appear only days or weeks after the vaccine has been given and their level falls gradually thereafter so that for some (e.g. those against the typhoid bacillus) it is necessary to repeat the dose of vaccine every few years. In the face of immediate risk of an active infection the antibodies are formed too slowly to be useful but in a few instances this difficulty may be overcome by injecting the person at risk with the serum of an animal which has been immunized. A horse injected with diphtheria toxoid develops antibodies in the same way as man. Blood serum from this horse will give a short period of immunity to a susceptible person (i.e. who has neither had diphtheria nor been immunized against it) if he is exposed to the risk of diphtheritic infection. Because most children have been immunized against diphtheria this method of protection is seldom used nowadays but it has a place in the treatment of a patient suffering from the disease.

4.3 Some general factors which influence infection

What is known of the cellular and humoral defences of the body is not enough to explain the distribution of infectious disease in the community. Personal experience suggests that some people are more subject to infectious disease than others. What follows is an attempt to describe some of the factors which make us more or less likely to acquire a parasite. The reasons for many of these factors are obscure.

The young and the old are more susceptible to infection than those of intermediate age. The reason for this is not clear and there are exceptions. Some viral infections, as, for example, yellow fever, which cause serious and often fatal disease in adults seem to produce only a mild infection in the young. It is a rare disease among adults native to the countries where it is seen because they are protected by an unnoticed attack which has occurred in childhood. Old age is, of course, associated with many disabilities and chronic diseases and it is not easy to separate the effects of these from age itself as factors in the encouragement of infectious diseases. The very young on the other hand seem to develop some of their natural antibodies slowly and, in fact, there are a very few people who never do so. Sooner or later these unfortunates are likely to die of some infectious disease. It is possible that the child 'who always has a cold' is to some extent less well endowed than his fellows with antibodies derived from experience but there is no real evidence of this.

There are no reliable grounds for thinking that the man in perfect condition, the trained athlete, is less liable to infection than his fellows. It is the company which he keeps, the possible sources of alien parasites, which determines the likelihood of infection.

Famine and pestilence have long been linked with human misery. A deficiency of protein in the diet interferes with the production of antibodies and may have other deleterious effects. Tuberculous infection which seems to be cured may be reactivated by a shortage of food. Kwashiorkor, a disease due to protein deficiency seen in many parts of Africa, is associated with increased susceptibility to many common infectious diseases. The death rate from measles in Zambia may be as high as 30% whereas in London it is less than 1%. A deficiency of some vitamins is another factor which encourages infectious disease but the mechanism of this is unknown. The effects of cold and fatigue can seldom be separated but both tend to reactivate quiescent infections. In the German concentration camps death was due, not to the major epidemic diseases such as typhus or relapsing fever, but to common diseases, bronchitis and boils, in an abnormally severe form. The victims had 'no resistance' which meant that the normal defensive mechanisms of their bodies had ceased to work.

Sudden fluctuations of atmospheric temperature and humidity as in passing from an over-heated house to freezing cold outside are thought to make the mucous membranes of the nose and throat more susceptible to viral infection. Experience suggests that we are most comfortable and suffer from fewer nasal infections at a steady temperature. There is not much evidence that the, to us, excessive heat of the tropics makes a man more susceptible to infectious disease. Many of the so-called 'tropical diseases' are limited to hot climates only because they are spread by insect vectors which cannot survive elsewhere.

There can be little doubt that the hormonal balance of the body influences parasitic infection. It was mentioned that the vagina of a woman of child-bearing age is protected from bacterial infection by its acidity. The oestrogenic hormone which she secretes at this stage of her life mobilizes the glycogen in the vaginal epithelium which is then converted to lactic acid by the action of the normal bacterial flora of the vagina. When the hormone is no longer secreted the pH of the vagina rises to 7·0 when bacterial infection is possible. Diabetes mellitus, caused by the failure of the pancreatic glands to secret insulin, increases the victim's liability to tuberculosis and staphylococcal boils. It has been suggested that this is due to the replacement of the lactic acid found in normal tissues by acetoacetic acid which is not inhibitory to bacteria. The hormones of the adrenal gland and the synthetic drugs with a similar action have a profound effect upon infection. In large doses these substances suppress the formation of antibodies and depress the defensive mechanisms of the body. Since many of the painful or harmful sequels to infection are due to an overaction of the defensive mechanisms these drugs play a useful part in medicine but there is always a risk that they will exacerbate an existing infection or stir up a quiescent one. This has been seen repeatedly in patients suffering from tuberculosis.

The nature of a man's work and especially his contact with some poisonous substances may affect his susceptibility to infectious disease. Silica dust, inhaled by miners and quarrymen, not only produces specific damage to the lungs (silicosis) but encourages tuberculous infection. Minor scratches caused by cadmium alloys (used in aircraft construction) are liable to infection: cadmium is a poisonous metal. X-rays and some substances such as benzene interfere with the cellular reactions of the body. Certain trades carry risk of infection because they involve work with substances which are likely to contain pathogenic bacteria: bone meal, made by pulverizing dry bones imported from India or East Africa, has caused anthrax in those who operate the grinding plant.

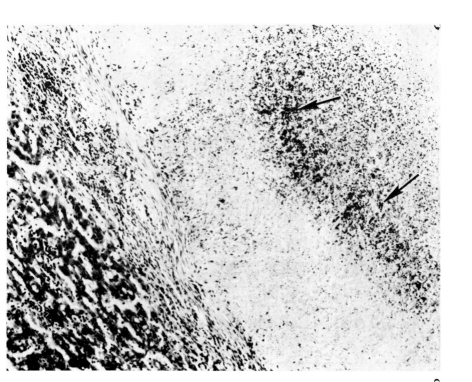

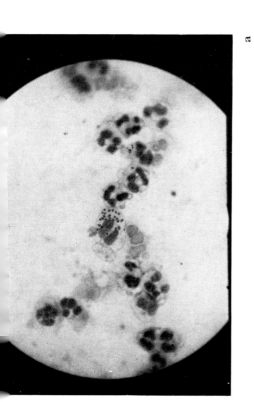

Plate 3 (a) Gonococci in pus. (×1000) (By courtesy of Dr. A. E. Wilkinson)

(b) Staphylococcal abscess of liver. (×350) (By courtesy of Lady Florey)

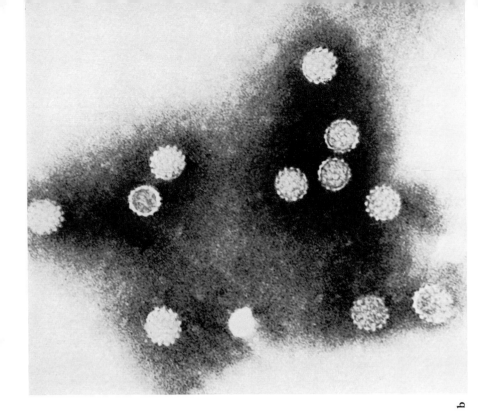

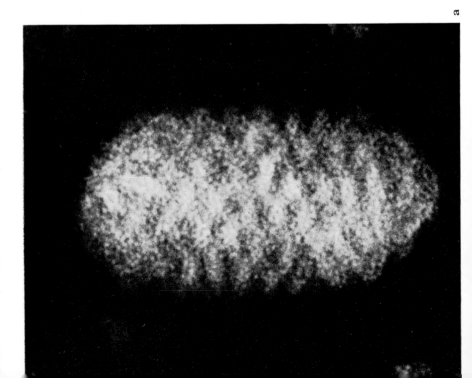

a

b

Localization and general effects of Disease   5

5.1 The localization of disease

It may well be asked why a streptococcus causes tonsillitis and a dysentery bacillus diarrhoea and not vice versa. We can only guess the answer. Every specific parasite has its own habits and habitat. The route by which it enters the body may play a part in deciding the site of multiplication but not very much. A staphylococcus entering the skin will usually confine its life in the host to the immediate neighbourhood of the point of entry. An anthrax bacillus entering by the same route will ultimately spread to the blood stream and throughout the body. Dysentery bacilli swallowed in food or drink multiply in the lumen of the bowel and nowhere else. The typhoid bacilli taken by the same route pass from the intestinal tract to the tissues and at a later stage of the disease return to the bowel. The gonococcus is usually confined to the genital tract: rarely it may invade the eyes or the joints of the skeleton but no other site. Streptococci are not really specific parasites. Most often they cause tonsillitis but they may infect the ear or the skin and from any of these sites may overflow into the blood. A streptococcus discharged by a patient with tonsillitis may cause some quite different infection in its next victim.

A parasite depends on its host for nutrition and it is reasonable to suppose that each establishes itself and succeeds best in that part of the body which best supplies its needs. By growing bacteria *in vitro* much has been learned of the conditions most suitable for the growth of individual parasites. Some bacteria demand only a simple mixture of peptones (or other breakdown products of proteins) with a carbohydrate and some sodium chloride. Others are more exigent and will not grow without several factors derived from blood. It is rarely that these requirements can be translated exactly into the conditions which prevail in the living body. The anaerobic bacteria which cause tetanus or gas gangrene can multiply only in an environment where the local oxygen tension is low. Their multiplication is limited to the deeper parts of wounds from which the oxygen supply has been cut off by damage to the surrounding tissues and by the exhaustion of the available oxygen by aerobic bacteria. A typical site would be the severe mangled wound caused in a road accident or a deep puncture by a thorn. The yeast-like fungi can multiply in an environment so acid that it prevents the multiplication of the common pathogenic bacteria. If the pH rises the fungi disappear: presumably they cannot compete for nutriments with the bacteria. A third example points to a more exact biochemical demands. *Brucella abortus* is a bacterium which causes contagious abortion in cows. In these animals it is localized to the mammae and the genital tract, and is excreted in the milk and vaginal discharges. Rarely it is transmitted to man in whom it causes a prolonged feverish illness: it is not localized but seems to persist in the liver, spleen and bone marrow, sometimes overflowing into the blood. (There is no obvious exit from these sites so that when the parasite has entered man it has come to the end of its parasitic life.) It has been found that *in vitro* the alcohol erythritol, while not essential for the growth of the parasite, encourages its multiplication. In nature erythritol is a rare substance which in man is distributed very sparsely throughout the body. In the cow it is concentrated in the genital tract and mammae and nowhere else. Such well-documented examples of bacterial localization are rare but it is a reasonable guess that what decides the site of a parasite within the host is the exact satisfaction of its nutritional needs. It is our ignorance of the life of the parasite *in vivo* which forbids more precise statements on this subject.

5.2   Some general effects of infectious disease

Experience tells us that infectious disease may take an almost infinite variety of forms both subjectively and objectively. There is no part of the body which will not nourish some parasite. Each species of parasite has its peculiar habits and effects. In one host a parasite will provoke a violent reaction and in another a trivial one. All (or almost all), however, stimulate the host to produce a specific antibody and induce physiological changes in the host which are much the same whatever the parasite may be. Man is a homoiothermic animal whose body temperature remains constant at about 37 °C. Violent exercise may raise this to 40 °C and prolonged exposure to cold may lower it. A rise in the body temperature is also a well recognized reaction to many parasitic infections but the mechanism for this is not entirely clear. Some species of bacteria (but not all) will produce a rise in temperature if injected into the blood stream. The effect is not a direct one but seems to depend on the interaction of the bacteria with the leucocytes in the blood to form a 'pyrogen' which acts on the centre in the nervous system which controls the body temperature. Associated with the increase in temperature is a rise in the metabolic rate of the body: the blood circulates more quickly and the chemical processes of the body are accelerated. Other sequels to a rise in temperature are headache, lack of appetite and sometimes profuse sweating with a sensation of cold. It is not easy to guess what might be the functions of these responses to infection. The antigen-antibody reactions take place more rapidly at 42 °C than at 37 °C. The rate of multiplication of some viruses falls off as the temperature rises above 37 °C. A few species of bacteria (e.g. the gonococcus) are killed at 42 °C but the temperature of a patient with gonorrhoea seldom reaches this level.

Fever is not the only cause of headache. An infection of the membranes surrounding the brain (meningitis) causes acute pain due apparently to a local rise in pressure comparable to the pain caused by a boil in a site where there is no room for expansion of the inflammatory process between the skin and the bone. Such a local increase in pressure can hardly explain why acute tonsillitis can make the throat feel very sore. The soreness is very plain to the victim but examination of the throat reveals only that it is red and perhaps slightly swollen, the results presumably of the local reaction to the infection. Most epithelial surfaces are well supplied with sensory nerves and it may be that these are stimulated directly by the bacterial or viral invasion. If the infection progresses to the point that the epithelial cells are destroyed to form an ulcer this is usually more or less painless.

The colicky pains in the abdomen which accompany dysentery are due to unusual activity of the muscles of the bowel wall stimulated, directly or indirectly, by bacterial toxins. The function of such activity would seem to be to expel the parasites but the victim may be more conscious of the pain than of any effect produced by the parasite directly. There are many symptoms produced by infectious disease for which there is no adequate explanation: why a patient with tonsillitis should feel sick or why a healing boil itches. The interpretation of the patient's symptoms in terms of bodily function is the keystone of the physician's art, based as it is on tradition, observation, experience and experiment.

Many infections cause no signs or symptoms or ones so slight that the patient does not heed them. The only evidence that they have occurred is the appearance of a specific antibody by which they can be identified. In most epidemics some of those who seem to have escaped infection can be shown to have antibodies to the parasite which caused it.

Infectious Disease and the Community 6

It is impossible to forecast with certainty whether any individual will contract a specific infectious disease. When such a disease as influenza is rife some of those exposed to infection appear to escape it entirely. Others who have had no known contact with any source of infection will develop the disease in a severe form. Infection is a matter of probability and some of the factors which make it more or less likely have been discussed. It is possible to titrate the levels of antibody to some parasites in individuals and experience indicates that a sufficiently high level is a reasonable promise of immunity.

For most of us infectious disease is an exceptional experience: we remember (or our mothers remember) when we had measles or chickenpox. These specific infections occur typically in epidemic form. The word 'epidemic' has no quantitative value and is applied equally to 12 cases of measles in a school or 30 cases of typhoid fever in one town or 10 000 cases of influenza in the country as a whole. The essential feature of an epidemic is that all the cases are due to a single kind of parasite and form a series of apparently related simultaneous or consequent infections. No doubt every epidemic has an origin in a single case. In an epidemic of influenza it is improbable that the original source of the parasite will be detected except in such a small community as a school. The origin of an epidemic of typhoid fever, however, can often be traced to a single carrier of the disease. The community at risk may be the family or a single class at school or the whole school or the entire population. None of these is a closed community. One or more members of it will have contact with the outside world and it is from the outside that the epidemic is introduced. The father may acquire the parasite at his work and bring it home to spread it to all the family. At least as often a child will introduce a parasite acquired from his schoolmates. In the first week of term every boy in the class will make his contribution of the parasites which he has picked up in the holidays. Most of these will do no harm but if one of them spreads to his fellows the disease may overflow into the entire school. In the same way a visitor from elsewhere may introduce a fresh parasite into a community. In the course of a nation-wide epidemic the returns made by medical officers often show that a disease, such as influenza, begins in a single town and spreads thence to the whole country. Some epidemics are plainly due to parasites introduced from overseas.

Whether a parasite spreads epidemically in a community will depend essentially on the level of specific antibodies in the community as a whole. Excepting the antibodies to a parasite which is entirely foreign to the community (such as the measles virus in Fiji) the level of antibody will range from enough to give entire protection to some individuals to none at all in others. The more there are of the second type the more likely is an epidemic. Once an epidemic has begun the population may be divided into four classes:

(i) Those suffering from the disease in a typical form.
(ii) Those suffering from the disease in a form so slight as to be un-detected but who are nevertheless a source of infection to others.
(iii) Those who are immune to the disease either because they have been protected deliberately or have had the disease recently.
(iv) Those who are susceptible to the disease but not yet infected.

The more there are of classes (i), (ii) and (iv) the more rapidly the disease will spread: the more there are in class (iii) the less probable is a major epidemic. As the epidemic progresses those in classes (i) and (ii) will be transferred to class (iii). In theory an epidemic will end only when there are no more individuals in class (iv). The analogy of the fire is appropriate. A single match lights it and it continues to burn until all the fuel is consumed.

The features which distinguish one epidemic from another will depend on the habits of the parasite, on its ability to stimulate the formation of antibodies and their duration, and on the deliberate attempts which are made to bring it to an end. To these may be added the 'incubation period', i.e. the time between the parasitic invasion and the first signs of this in the patient. This time may range from less than 24 hours for the common cold to 14–21 days for typhoid fever. For any one disease it is constant within a few days. This interval does not change the pattern of epidemic disease but only its timetable. Some diseases are clearly more infectious than others: the numbers of parasites set free by the first host, their ability to survive outside the hosts and the route by which they re-enter a host are all factors in this. Few children exposed to measles or mumps for the first time escape infection. Diphtheria, which is also spread from the respiratory tract, is far less infectious while ringworm, spread by direct contact, is even less so. It has been observed in some large cities that measles is epidemic only in alternate years which suggests that epidemic spread will occur only when the natural increase of the population has provided a certain minimum of non-immunes. Epidemic diphtheria is rare in this country because, owing to deliberate immunization, there are not enough non-immunes: nevertheless sporadic cases of diphtheria are seen from time to time who would certainly initiate an epidemic in a less immune community.

Attempts to limit or terminate an epidemic may take several forms. The basis of most of them is to separate the sources of infection from those who are susceptible. The visitor to this country who develops smallpox which he has acquired overseas is isolated strictly and seen only by doctors and nurses who have been recently vaccinated against the disease. It is likely that before his disease has been recognized he has been shedding the virus for at least a few hours so that an attempt is made to trace those with whom he has been in contact. If found these too are isolated until it is certain that they are not incubating the disease. (Smallpox is not only a dangerous disease but a highly infectious one.) Suppose, however, that the person who introduces smallpox is partially immune to the disease: the effects of deliberate vaccination do not last for ever and he may not have been vaccinated since childhood. His disease may under these circumstances take a mild form not easily recognized as smallpox: he may not think it necessary to visit a doctor: it is unlikely that he will be isolated and he may spread his infection far and wide. It is possible that he will never be detected and his existence known of only from the appearance of typical smallpox in some of his contacts. A detailed study of the spread of measles and poliomyelitis makes it certain that the patient with mild or unrecognized symptoms plays a large part in spreading these diseases. The boy who has acute streptococcal tonsillitis will be kept away from school, or, if a boarder, will be isolated. The one with a mild sore throat caused by the same parasite attends and spreads his infection to his contacts. Some of his victims will be so ill that they are kept from school (class i): others less ill but equally likely to spread streptococci will stay at school (class ii). The process will continue until there are no more susceptibles (class iv) at risk. In practice it is often found that the originator of the epidemic is a boy who suffers from a chronic streptococcal infection, perhaps of the ear, who never shows any symptoms of a sore throat (class ii). A laboratory examination will detect all those who harbour streptococci whether they are ill or not and the exclusion from school of all these carriers should end the epidemic. Unfortunately any laboratory examination takes a day or two so that while it is in progress the disease may have spread further.

Another method of dealing with an epidemic in such a community as a school is to attempt to isolate not the sources of infection but the potential victims. If the majority are clearly suffering from the disease it may be less inconvenient to isolate the uninfected minority. Since their isolation will rob them of any chance of acquiring a natural immunity they must not be readmitted to the community until it is certain that there are no more sources of infection.

Yet another method of ending an epidemic is to treat the whole community, sick and well, with a drug such as an antibiotic to eradicate the parasite. Whatever its advantages on paper this has not been very successful in practice and there are strong arguments against using powerful drugs except in the cure of apparent disease. However immediately distressing a disease may be, so long as it carries no serious risk to health it may be wiser to make no attempt to isolate the sources of infection but to hope that all those who are susceptible will acquire the infection and subsequent immunity as soon as possible. Many mothers take no steps to shield their children from such mild diseases as German measles: the immunity lasts for ever and 'it is better to get it over'. Recent research has shown that this is sound policy at any rate for girls: German measles in pregnancy is liable to cause deformities in the unborn child. It is difficult to exclude all infectious pupils from a school. It is almost impossible to keep infectious adults from a larger community. Even before microscopic parasites were recognized as a cause of disease it was suspected that the visitor from outside was responsible for epidemics. When plague flourished in the Turkish empire the western nations used to establish a 'quarantine' at their frontiers where the incoming traveller was forced to wait for forty days (as the name suggests). The scheme was not satisfactory. Certain classes of travellers and those who gave rewards in the right quarter were not detained. When cholera spread from India to continental Europe at least three times in the nineteenth century a quarantine was established to prevent its further spread to the British Isles and the USA. It failed and both countries suffered transient but destructive epidemics.

Cholera is a waterborne disease. Its spread is largely due to the pollution of drinking water by human faeces. Nowadays it seldom spreads to any country with modern sewerage and adequate supplies of pure water. The implications of waterborne disease are not quite the same as those of a disease spread by aerial routes or direct contact. Since most waterborne parasites will survive for some days in that medium the hazards of transfer from one host to another are less and infection is more certain. It is characteristic that a large number, perhaps all, of the susceptibles among those who drink the infected water will acquire the infection more or less simultaneously. Infection by an aerial route is likely to be a continuous process as each victim becomes in turn a further source of infection. Waterborne infections are now rare in Great Britain and such as do occur are almost always the result of an accident: the automatic chlorinating plant fails or a water main is cracked (from age or the weight of traffic above it) to allow the ingress of pollution. The most serious waterborne disease in the British Isles is typhoid fever which, though usually spread from a human carrier by water or milk, may be passed directly from man to man. In countries where water liable to faecal pollution is used for all domestic purposes large epidemics of the disease are rare because many of the population have some degree of immunity derived from experience of the disease but casual infections are not uncommon. Foodborne epidemics show a timetable similar to that of those spread by water. All susceptibles who eat the food acquire infection simultaneously: those who do not eat the infected food escape. By comparing the diet of the two groups it is often possible to identify the source of infection at once.

The majority of epidemic diseases seen in the British Isles will be those to which some part of those exposed to them will have a total or partial immunity. In very few epidemics—even waterborne ones—will all those at risk acquire infection. A possible exception is the so-called 'winter vomiting disease' which may cause a trivial and short-lived epidemic of nausea and vomiting in almost all the pupils of a school within a few hours.

It has many of the characteristics of a water- or foodborne disease but intensive search has failed to reveal a parasitic cause. It seems most likely that it is caused by an airborne virus of high infectivity which produces a very short-lived immunity. It is the parasite recently introduced to a community or one which is in process of adapting itself to a parasitic life which is likely to find most susceptible hosts. For many years measles was unknown in Greenland but when it was introduced in 1935 99% of the population was infected. The Black Death, which was almost certainly plague introduced from overseas, is thought to have killed about a quarter of the population of the British Isles in the fourteenth century. It is not easy to find an example of a parasite which is in the process of adapting itself to man as a host, but the patterns of human disease change. There is some evidence that the influenza epidemic which ravaged the entire world in 1917–18 was caused by a virus derived from pigs. One form of dysentery now common in this country was not recognized before 1933: the severity of the disease has not changed but whereas at first it was a disease of the late summer it is now most frequent in the winter. Syphilis was first recognized in Europe at the end of the fifteenth century as an acute and painful disease; in the course of time it has become a chronic and painless (but lethal) one. These instances do no more than suggest that adjustment of a micro-organism to a parasitic existence in man is a slow process which may involve a change in its habits and its effects on man. There is no reason for believing that other micro-organisms may not at some date in the future exchange a free-living existence or a parasitic life in animals for one in which they draw their nutriments from man.

It is sometimes suggested that some races or groups of man are more or less susceptible to specific infections than the rest of the human race. It has been noticed for many years that the young Irish of both sexes seem especially liable to infectious disease when they migrate to London. There are no figures to support this thesis but coming as many of them do from thinly populated rural areas they probably lack the antibodies of experience which are common in our urban populations. In the same way there has been some alarm at the number of Pakistanis who enter this country suffering from tuberculosis. It is not generally realized that in all the less favoured parts of the world where overcrowding and malnutrition are frequent tuberculosis is the major infectious disease. Given modern medical treatment it is, however, a curable one and there seems to be no reason to fear that imported tuberculosis is a grave threat to our public health. Some people have argued that Jews are less liable to tuberculosis than Gentiles because after generations spent in overcrowded and insanitary ghettoes natural selection has eliminated the lines of the race which are more susceptible to the disease. There is no real evidence for this thesis but the idea is an interesting one.

There are some diseases, usually labelled collectively as 'tropical diseases', which are naturally limited to the warmer parts of the world.

The reasons for this localization are various. Many are spread from host to host by blood-sucking insects which cannot survive in temperate climates. Malaria which a few years ago probably claimed more victims than any other infectious disease is caused by a protozoon which shares its parasitic life between man and mosquito. In many countries DDT and other modern insecticides have eradicated the mosquito and thereby broken the parasitic cycle. This has been one of the most important advances in preventive medicine in the last thirty years. There are, however, at least four species of mosquito to be found in Great Britain which can act as host to the malaria parasite and native malaria persisted in the marshes of Kent and Essex until about 1920 and there was a minor outbreak in London in 1952. Yellow fever, which can be prevented by vaccination, survives in Central America because the virus can use monkeys as a host alternative to man. Many waterborne diseases flourish in the tropics not because of the climate but by reasons of the low standards of hygiene which prevail. History has shown that it is only our pure water supplies and efficient sewerage which protects us from the spread of epidemic cholera.

Parasites Transmitted to Man from Animals

The discussion so far has been restricted to the parasites which spread from one human host to another. There are, however, some bacteria, viruses and fungi which are normally parasitic on animals but which may on occasion exchange their normal host for man. This happens infrequently and most of those who acquire disease from animals are those, such as veterinary surgeons and farmers, who have close contact with animals. Infection by *Brucella abortus* has been mentioned previously. It is a highly infectious disease of cows causing them to lose their first or second calves and responsible for considerable financial loss to the farmer. Man acquires the parasite either by drinking milk from an infected cow or from her vaginal discharges when she is calving. (Pasteurization renders the milk safe for human consumption.) The spread of the parasite from man to man or man to cow is unknown since it is not excreted by the human host.

Anthrax is a fatal disease which may attack almost any animal. Because the anthrax bacillus forms spores it can persist almost indefinitely in dust, on pasture contaminated by an infected animal or in such animal products as bone meal (used in feeding stuffs and as a fertilizer) if these have been made from the carcass of an infected animal. Man acquires the parasite either from these or other animal products or from close contact with an infected animal which may discharge the parasite in milk, faeces or shed blood. If untreated the parasite in both animals and man is likely to invade the entire body and will probably cause death. It is said that some species of birds which feed on carrion are immune to anthrax: if this is so it is an interesting example of evolutionary resistance to infectious disease. Orf (in the west of England, 'lure') is a viral disease of sheep which causes chronic ulcers of the skin when it is transmitted to man by direct contact. Cowpox has been mentioned before. It may be transmitted from cow to man and vice versa by direct contact and in man is a far less serious disease than smallpox although closely related antigenically. Ringworm caught from animals is caused by several species of fungi which are distinct from those which cause strictly human ringworm. They provoke an acute reaction in the human skin in contrast to the milder but more persistent reaction caused by fungi of human origin. Fifty years ago tuberculosis derived from drinking milk from tuberculous cows was a major problem in public health. The tubercle bacilli responsible are distinct from but closely related to those which may spread from man to man. Bovine tuberculosis is now almost extinct since the disease has been eradicated from the cattle population by a vigorous policy of detection and slaughter of the infected animals. Among the diseases caught from animals tuberculosis was exceptional in that the parasite could occasionally pass from man to cows.

Plague has been the cause of some of the more devastating human epidemics but it is naturally an endemic disease of rodents. Marked fluctuations in their numbers is a phenomenon noticed in many rodent species (rats, field mice, lemmings) and is often accompanied by the appearance of epidemic diseases among them which may play some part in reducing their numbers. Plague survives as a sporadic disease in several species of wild rodents in northern India, South Africa and California. When from time to time there is a marked increase in the numbers of domestic rats epidemic plague may appear among them. From them the bacillus is carried to man by the bite of a flea and kills about half those infected. There is no climatic reason why plague should not flourish in Europe but here there are no reservoirs of plague in wild rodents and man seldom lives in close proximity to rats. Plague is a disease of the slums but at the time of the Great Plague (1665) most of the inhabitants of London lived in what we would now think of as filthy slums. At that time the brown rat (*R. norwegicus*) had not yet displaced the black rat (*R. rattus*) which, because it is a more domestic animal, is more usually the source of human plague.

These are a few of the diseases which man may acquire from animals. Few of them spread from man to man or from man to animals which suggests that they are ill-adapted to a parasitic life in man but this may not be a complete explanation. Bovine tuberculosis and cowpox can both spread from man to cows. There would seem no reason why anthrax should not do the same but a man with an anthrax infection of his hand, a so-called 'malignant pustule', is unlikely to shake hands with his friends or handle his animals. It may be a lack of ability to spread which makes invasion of man a dead-end for most of these parasites. There are, however, a few parasites (e.g. the gonococcus) which are found only in man and others, common in animals, which infect man rarely. For each of the higher plants there is an environment in which it flourishes best; in another environment it survives; in yet another it will not grow at all. There may be a parallel among the smaller parasites.

There is one genus of bacteria which includes many species which appear to be equally at home in man and a variety of animals. *Salmonella* includes species which are strictly specific in their choice of hosts: *S. typhi* (causing typhoid fever) is limited to man and *S. pullorum* to chicks. Most of the species, however, appear to be equally at home in man and animals. They commonly enter man in his food or drink producing diarrhoea and vomiting and are the commonest cause of 'food poisoning'. The food may be meat derived from an animal which was infected when it was slaughtered or milk drawn from an infected cow. The infection is endemic in rats and mice which may contaminate the food in the larder with their droppings. But a cook or a waiter may equally well be the source of the infection if he is suffering from the disease not too severely. Most of the members of this genus seem to be well-adapted parasites able to live in a variety of environments and they can survive for some time in animal feeding stuffs (most of which contain meat residues) and sewage. It is not human infection which is remarkable but our relative freedom from infection.

CONCLUSION

Infectious disease in man is usually thought of as a danger which must be avoided or prevented. This book has tried to regard the problem as a special example of the phenomena of parasitism. Space has prevented the discussion of many of the aspects of the problem which deserve more detailed attention but when we get a cold it may amuse us to think of it not as a trivial but vexatious burden to our existence but an example of successful parasitism by an invisible virus.

Practical Work

1. Practical studies of the phenomena of infectious disease are not easy. Experimental work using man as a subject has obvious limitations although some of the pioneers of bacteriology performed the most hair-raising experiments on themselves and their colleagues. Much of our knowledge is derived from experiments on animals but these are subject to severe limitations by the Cruelty to Animals Act, 1883. It is a field better left to the medical profession.

2. There are no difficulties in demonstrating some bacterial parasites and in growing them *in vitro*. Even if it is impossible to isolate any parasite which is causing disease the gross appearance and habits of those which live symbiotically on the surfaces on man are not greatly different from the pathogenic organisms. An even greater variety of bacteria may be found in such substances as 'ripe' cheese or in the trap of a kitchen sink. Because of their size all these bacteria must be examined microscopically under the 1/12 in. objective but except for this most of the apparatus can be improvised. To grow bacteria *in vitro* the main requirements are suitable culture media and a thermostatically controlled incubator to maintain 37 °C for human material. Many non-parasitic bacteria will flourish at lower temperatures. Admirable directions for the examination of bacteria are to be found in *School Microbiology*, Oxoid Ltd, Southwark Bridge Road, London, SE1. For those who wish to pursue the subject further the following book will give all the information needed.
COLLINS, C. H. and PATRICIA LYNE. *Microbiological Methods.* (1970). Butterworths, London.

3. It may be possible to demonstrate some of the factors which influence the spread of infection by the collection of statistics within the class or school. Since it is clearly undesirable that the nature of any pupil's illness should be common knowledge such a study must be limited to observable phenomena such as absence from school on the grounds of ill-health. If the number of those absent is plotted graphically against time it may be possible to show an increase in the first weeks of term while newly introduced parasites are being spread among those unused to them: in a boarding school it may be that such a ceremony as Speech Day will have a similar effect owing to the number of strangers who have entered the community. It would be a matter of some interest to know how the incidence of infectious disease among the fittest members of the community (e.g. the 1st and 2nd XVs) compares with that in the less athletic. If 1/10 in. graph paper is used one small square on the horizontal scale might represent 1 day and on the vertical scale 1 person: the general effect is seen in Fig. 3–1.

Statistical studies are not of great value unless the total numbers are large. The whole school provides better material than a single class and, with the cooperation of the education authority, it might be possible to study the records of absence from all the schools in a town.

Some of the parasites mentioned in this book

Bacteria	Portal of entry	Site of localization
Staphylococcus	Skin	Site of entry or anywhere in the tissues
Streptococcus	Respiratory tract or skin	Site of entry or anywhere in the tissues
Gonococcus	Genital tract	Genital tract
Pneumococcus	Respiratory tract	Lungs
Diphtheria bacillus	Respiratory tract	Throat
Escherichia coli	?	Urinary tract
Typhoid bacillus	Mouth	Spleen, etc.
Salmonella spp.	Mouth	Intestine
Dysentery bacillus	Mouth	Intestine
Anthrax bacillus	Skin	Skin and whole body

Fungi		
Ringworm	Skin	Skin

Viruses		
Common cold	Respiratory Tract	Nose
Influenza	Respiratory tract	Respiratory tract
Measles	Respiratory tract	Respiratory tract and skin
Smallpox	Respiratory tract	Skin
Polio virus	Intestine	Nervous system
Wart	Skin	Skin

Further Reading

BROCKINGTON, FRAZER (1958). *World Health*, Pelican, Harmondsworth, Middlesex.

BURNET, F. M. (1953). *Viruses and Man*, Pelican, Harmondsworth, Middlesex.

DUBOS, R. J. (1965). *Man Adapting*, Yale Univ. Press, New Haven. A diffuse but readable book by one of the greatest living scholars of infectious disease but also dealing with other problems of man's position in his environment.

DUBOS, R. J. (1970). *Man, Medicine and Environment*, Pelican, Harmondsworth, Middlesex.

DUBOS, R. J. and DUBOS, J. (1952). *The White Plague: tuberculosis, man and society*, Gollancz, London, 1952. A history of tuberculosis.

GALE, A. H. (1959). *Epidemic Diseases*, Pelican, Harmondsworth, Middlesex.

LAPAGE, G. (1957). *Animals Parasitic in Man*, Pelican, Harmondsworth, Middlesex.

TURK, D. C. and PORTER, I. A. (1965). *Short Textbook of Microbiology*, English Universities Press, London. A modern, accurate and compact textbook of human microbiology (which includes bacteria viruses and fungi).

ZINNSER, H. (1942). *Rats, Lice and History*, Routledge, London. The effects of infectious disease and (in particular) typhus fever on human history.